Air Fryer Breakfast Collection

The Ultimate Air Fryer Cookbook for your Breakfast

Lydia Gorman

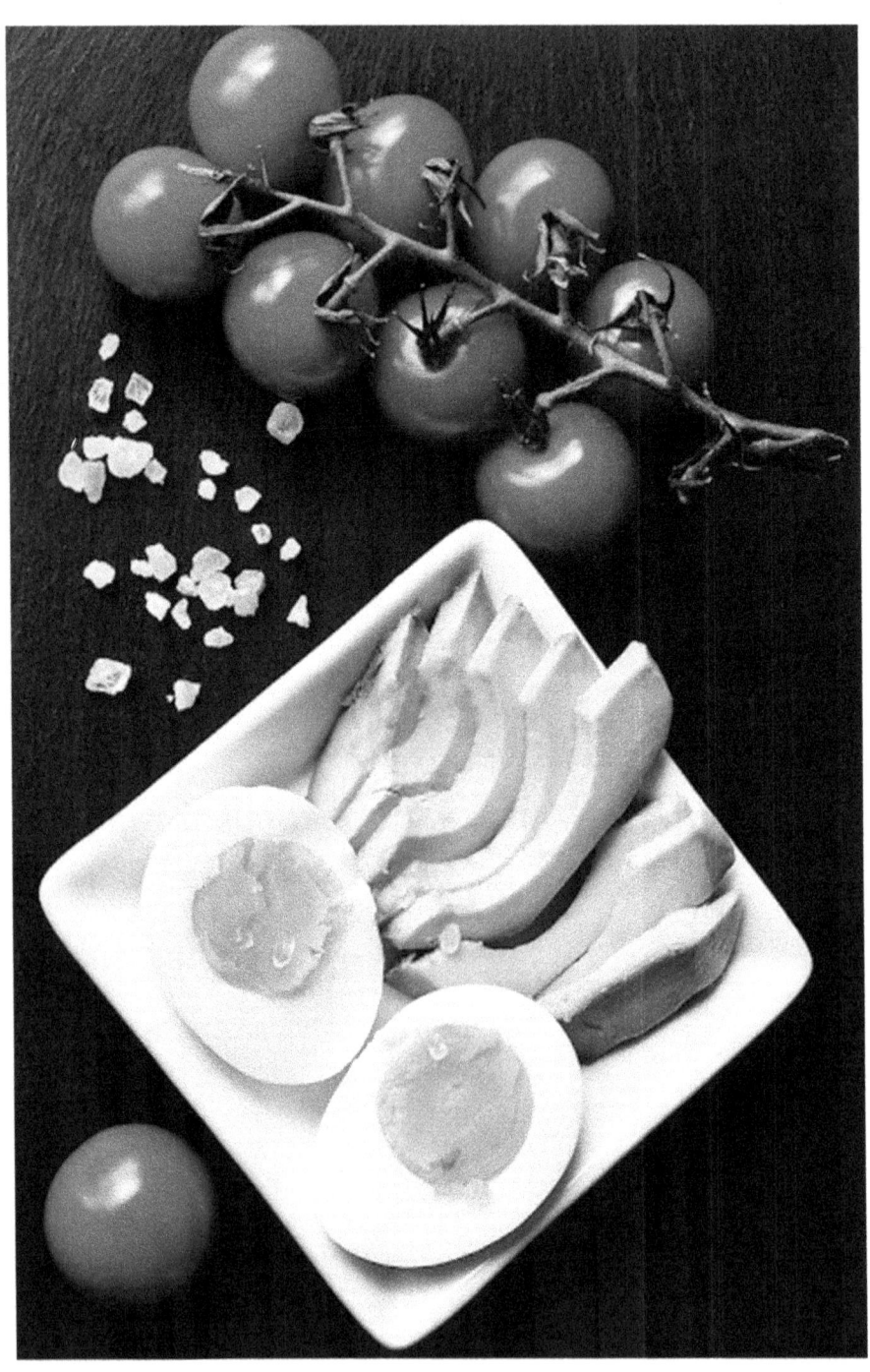

© Copyright 2020 All rights reserved.

The following Book is reproduced below with the goal of providing information that is as accurate and reliable as possible. Regardless, purchasing this Book can be seen as consent to the fact that both the publisher and the author of this book are in no way experts on the topics discussed within and that any recommendations or suggestions that are made herein are for entertainment purposes only. Professionals should be consulted as needed prior to undertaking any of the action endorsed herein.

This declaration is deemed fair and valid by both the American Bar Association and the Committee of Publishers Association and is legally binding throughout the United States.

Furthermore, the transmission, duplication, or reproduction of any of the following work including specific information will be considered an illegal act irrespective of

if it is done electronically or in print. This extends to creating a secondary or tertiary copy of the work or a recorded copy and is only allowed with the express written consent from the Publisher. All additional right reserved.

The information in the following pages is broadly considered a truthful and accurate account of facts and as such, any inattention, use, or misuse of the information in question by the reader will render any resulting actions solely under their purview. There are no scenarios in which the publisher or the original author of this work can be in any fashion deemed liable for any hardship or damages that may befall them after undertaking information described herein.

Additionally, the information in the following pages is intended only for informational purposes and should thus be thought of as universal. As befitting its nature, it is presented without assurance regarding its prolonged validity or interim quality. Trademarks that are mentioned are done without written consent and can in no way be considered an endorsement from the trademark holder.

Table of Contents

CHEESE EGG QUICHE 10

CHORIZO CASSEROLE 12

SAUSAGE EGG OMELET 14

CHEESE HAM EGG MUFFINS 16

PERFECT BAKED OMELET 18

BROCCOLI CASSEROLE 21

ZUCCHINI BREAD 23

EGG BITES 25

SPINACH SAUSAGE EGG MUFFINS 27

CHEESE PEPPER EGG BAKE 29

ALMOND BROCCOLI MUFFINS 31

ITALIAN BREAKFAST FRITTATA 33

FRESH HERB EGG CUPS 35

FETA PEPPER EGG MUFFINS 37

VANILLA RASPBERRY MUFFINS 39

BREAKFAST BAKE EGG 41

EASY CHICKEN EGG CUPS 43

EASY BREAKFAST SAUSAGE 45

ZUCCHINI BREAKFAST CASSEROLE 48

BASIL CHEESE ZUCCHINI QUICHE 50

ASPARAGUS QUICHE	52
MOIST PUMPKIN MUFFINS	54
HEALTHY ZUCCHINI GRATIN	56
ARTICHOKE QUICHE	59
TOMATO FETA FRITTATA	61
BLUEBERRY CREAM CHEESE TOASTS	63
ONION & CHEDDAR OMELET	65
SPICY EGG & BACON TORTILLA WRAPS	66
TURKEY & MUSHROOM SANDWICH	67
GRILLED TOFU SANDWICH WITH CABBAGE	69
OMELET BREAD CUPS	71
PROSCIUTTO, MOZZARELLA & EGGS IN A CUP	73
CRUSTLESS MEDITERRANEAN QUICHE	75
AIR FRIED ITALIAN CALZONE	77
ITALIAN SAUSAGE PATTIES	79
BRIOCHE TOAST WITH CHOCOLATE	80
BREAKFAST EGG MUFFINS WITH SHRIMP	82
KIWI MUFFINS WITH PECANS	84
HEARTY BANANA PASTRY	86
MANGO BREAD	87
PUMPKIN & SULTANAS' BREAD	89
FRENCH TOAST WITH VANILLA FILLING	91

GREEK-STYLE FRITTATA 93

MORNING POTATO SKINS 96

BUTTERED EGGS IN HOLE 98

LOADED EGG PEPPER RINGS 100

CHILI HASH BROWNS 101

JAPANESE-STYLE OMELET 103

BAKED KALE OMELET 105

BAKED AVOCADO WITH EGGS & CILANTRO 106

Introduction

What's the difference between an air fryer and deep fryer? Air fryers bake food at a high temperature with a high-powered fan, while deep fryers cook food in a vat of oil that has been heated up to a specific temperature. Both cook food quickly, but an air fryer requires practically zero preheat time while a deep fryer can take upwards of 10 minutes. Air fryers also require little to no oil and deep fryers require a lot that absorb into the food. Food comes out crispy and juicy in both appliances, but don't taste the same, usually because deep fried foods are coated in batter that cook differently in an air fryer vs a deep fryer. Battered foods needs to be sprayed with oil before cooking in an air fryer to help them color and get crispy, while the hot oil soaks into the batter in a deep fryer. Flour-based batters and wet batters don't cook well in an air fryer, but they come out very well in a deep fryer.

The ketogenic diet is one such example. The diet calls for a very small number of carbs to be eaten. This means food such as rice, pasta, and other starchy vegetables like potatoes are off the menu. Even relaxed versions of the keto diet minimize carbs to a large extent and this compromises the goals of many dieters. They end up having to exert large amounts of willpower to follow the diet. This doesn't do them any favors since willpower is like a muscle. At some point, it tires and this is when the dieter goes right back to their old pattern of eating. I have personal experience with this. In terms of health benefits, the keto diet offers the most. The reduction of carbs forces your body to mobilize fat and this results in automatic fat loss and better health.

Feel free to mix and match the recipes you see in here and play around with them. Eating is supposed to be fun! Unfortunately, we've associated fun eating with unhealthy food. This doesn't have to be the case. The air fryer, combined with the Mediterranean diet, will make your mealtimes fun-filled again and full of taste. There's no grease and messy cleanups to deal with anymore. Are you excited yet?

You should be! You're about to embark on a journey full of air fried goodness!

Cheese Egg Quiche

Preparation Time: 10 minutes

Cooking Time: 45 minutes

Serve: 6

Ingredients

8 eggs 6 oz cheddar cheese shredded

5 tbsp butter melted

6 oz cream cheese

Directions

Add eggs, cheese, butter, and cream cheese into the mixing bowl and blend using a hand mixer until well combined.

Pour egg mixture into the greased pie dish.

Cover dish with foil.

Select Bake mode.

Set time to 45 minutes and temperature 325 F then press START.

The air fryer display will prompt you to ADD FOOD once the temperature is reached then place the pie dish in the air fryer basket. Serve and enjoy.

Chorizo Casserole

Preparation Time: 10 minutes

Cooking Time: 55 minutes

Serve: 6

Ingredients

8 eggs

1 cup cheddar cheese shredded

1 bell pepper diced

4 oz can green chiles drained and chopped

3/4 cup heavy cream

1/2 lb ground chorizo sausage

1/4 tsp pepper

1/2 tsp salt

Directions

Cook chorizo in a pan over medium-high heat for 8 minutes or until browned.

In a bowl, whisk eggs with cream, pepper, and salt.

Stir in cooked chorizo, cheese, bell pepper, and green chiles.

Pour egg mixture into the greased baking dish.

Cover dish with foil.

Select Bake mode.

Set time to 40 minutes and temperature 350 F then press START.

The air fryer display will prompt you to ADD FOOD once the temperature is reached then place the baking dish in the air fryer basket.

Serve and enjoy.

Sausage Egg Omelet

Preparation Time: 10 minutes

Cooking Time: 30 minutes

Serve: 12

Ingredients

7 eggs

1 lb breakfast sausage

1 tsp mustard

3/4 cup heavy whipping cream

1/4 onion chopped

2 cups cheddar cheese shredded

1/2 bell pepper chopped

1/4 tsp pepper

1/2 tsp salt

Directions

Add sausage into the pan and cook until brown, add onion and bell pepper and cook for 2 minutes.

In a bowl, whisk eggs with 1 1/2 cups cheddar cheese, cream, mustard, pepper, and salt.

Stir in sausage mixture.

Pour egg mixture into the greased 9*13-inch baking dish.

Top with remaining cheese.

Cover dish with foil.

Select Bake mode.

Set time to 20 minutes and temperature 350 F then press START.

The air fryer display will prompt you to ADD FOOD once the temperature is reached then place the baking dish in the air fryer basket.

Serve and enjoy.

Cheese Ham Egg Muffins

Preparation Time: 10 minutes

Cooking Time: 20 minutes

Serve: 12

Ingredients

12 eggs

1 3/4 cup cheddar cheese shredded

2 cups ham diced

1 tsp garlic minced

1/2 pepper

1/2 tsp salt

Directions

In a bowl, whisk eggs with garlic, pepper, and salt.

Stir in cheddar cheese and ham.

Pour egg mixture into the silicone muffin molds.

Select Bake mode.

Set time to 20 minutes and temperature 375 F then press START.

The air fryer display will prompt you to ADD FOOD once the temperature is reached then place muffin molds in the air fryer basket.

Serve and enjoy.

Perfect Baked Omelet

Preparation Time: 10 minutes

Cooking Time: 45 minutes

Serve: 6

Ingredients

8 eggs

1 cup bell pepper chopped

1/2 cup onion chopped

1/2 cup cheddar cheese shredded

6 oz cooked ham diced

1 cup unsweetened almond milk

1/2 tsp salt

Directions

In a bowl, whisk eggs with milk and salt.

Stir in bell pepper, onion, cheese, and ham.

Pour egg mixture into the greased 8-inch baking dish.

Select Bake mode.

Set time to 45 minutes and temperature 350 F then press START.

The air fryer display will prompt you to ADD FOOD once the temperature is reached then place the baking dish in the air fryer basket.

Serve and enjoy.

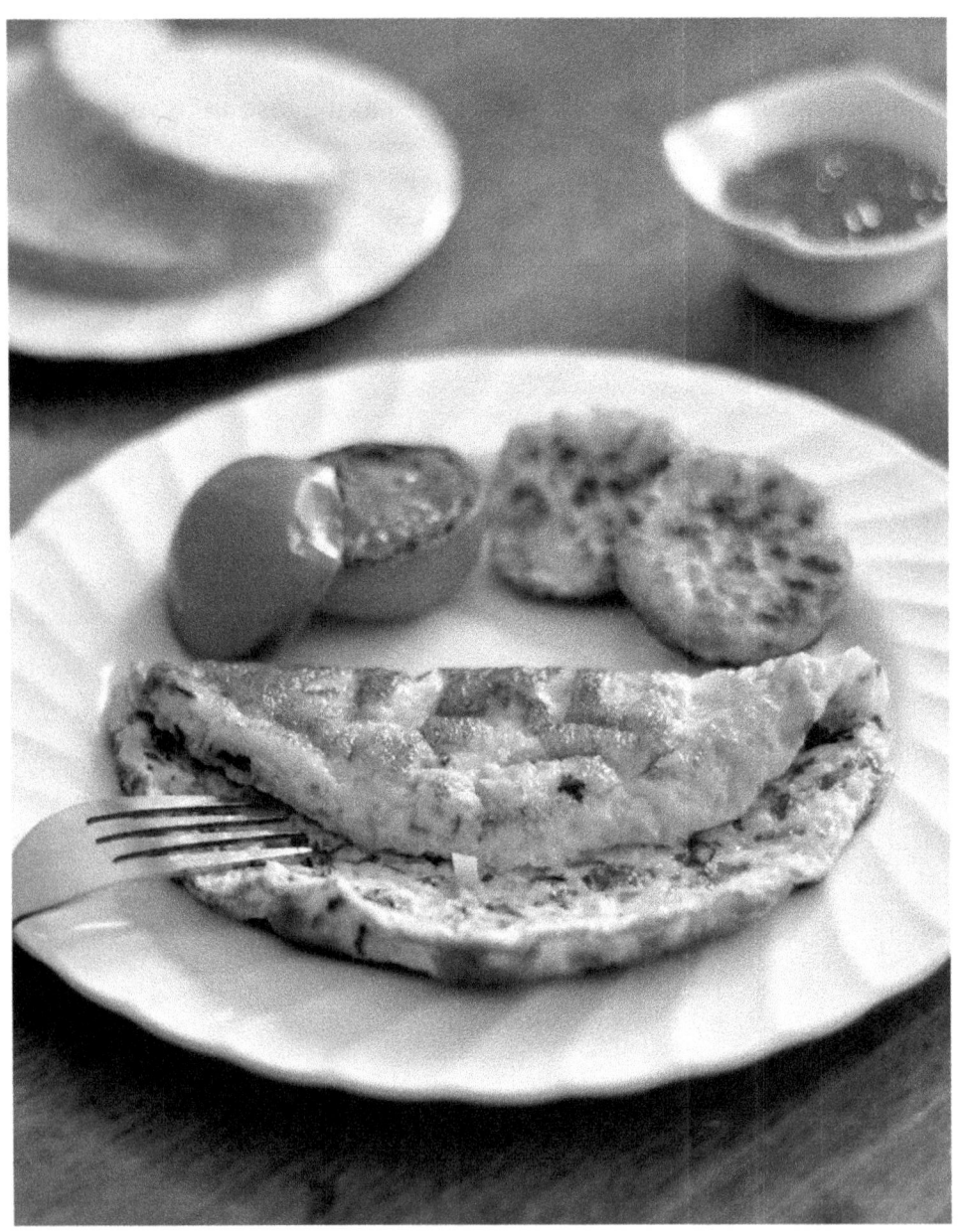

Broccoli Casserole

Preparation Time: 10 minutes

Cooking Time: 20 minutes

Serve: 4

Ingredients

2 cups broccoli florets chopped

1 cup cheddar cheese grated

1/2 cup sour cream

1/2 cup heavy cream

Pepper

Salt

Directions

In a bowl, whisk together heavy cream, sour cream, 1/2 cheddar cheese, pepper, and salt.

Add broccoli florets into the baking dish.

Pour heavy cream mixture over broccoli.

Top with remaining cheese.

Cover baking dish with foil.

Select Bake mode.

Set time to 20 minutes and temperature 350 F then press START.

The air fryer display will prompt you to ADD FOOD once the temperature is reached then place the baking dish in the air fryer basket.

Serve and enjoy

Zucchini Bread

Preparation Time: 10 minutes

Cooking Time: 60 minutes

Serve: 12

Ingredients

2 eggs, lightly beaten

1 1/2 cups zucchini grated

1/4 cup butter melted

1 tsp baking soda

1/2 cup erythritol

1/2 tsp ground cinnamon 2

 cups almond flour

1/2 tsp salt

Directions

In a small bowl, whisk together eggs and butter.

In a mixing bowl, mix together almond flour, cinnamon, sweetener, baking soda, and salt.

Add zucchini and egg mixture and mix until well combined.

Pour batter into the greased loaf pan.

Select Bake mode.

Set time to 60 minutes and temperature 350 F then press START.

The air fryer display will prompt you to ADD FOOD once the temperature is reached then place the loaf pan in the air fryer basket.

Slice and serve.

Egg Bites

Preparation Time: 10 minutes

Cooking Time: 10 minutes

Serve: 4

Ingredients

4 eggs 1/4 cup cheddar cheese shredded

4 bacon slices cooked and crumbled

1/2 bell pepper diced

1/2 onion diced

1 tbsp unsweetened almond milk

Pepper

Salt

Directions

In a bowl, whisk eggs with cheese, milk, pepper, and salt.

Stir in bacon, bell pepper, and onion.

Pour egg mixture into the 4 silicone muffin molds.

Select Air Fry mode.

Set time to 10 minutes and temperature 300 F then press START.

The air fryer display will prompt you to ADD FOOD once the temperature is reached then place muffin molds in the air fryer basket.

Serve and enjoy.

Spinach Sausage Egg Muffins

Preparation Time: 10 minutes

Cooking Time: 20 minutes

Serve: 6

Ingredients

2 eggs

5 egg whites

3 lean breakfast turkey sausage

1/4 cup cheddar cheese shredded

1/4 cup spinach chopped

1/4 cup unsweetened almond milk

Pepper

Salt

Directions

In a pan, brown the turkey sausage over medium-high heat until sausage is brown.

Cut sausage in small pieces and set aside.

In a bowl, whisk eggs, egg whites, milk, pepper, and salt.

Stir in spinach.

Pour egg mixture into the silicone muffin molds.

Divide sausage and cheese evenly between each muffin mold.

Select Bake mode.

Set time to 20 minutes and temperature 350 F then press START.

The air fryer display will prompt you to ADD FOOD once the temperature is reached then place muffin molds in the air fryer basket.

Serve and enjoy

Cheese Pepper Egg Bake

Preparation Time: 10 minutes

Cooking Time: 30 minutes

Serve: 2

Ingredients

3 eggs

1/2 cup cottage cheese

1 1/2 tbsp jalapeno chopped

1/2 cup pepper jack cheese shredded

1/8 tsp pepper

1/8 tsp sea salt

Directions

In a bowl, whisk eggs with pepper and salt.

Stir in jalapeno, pepper jack cheese, and cottage cheese.

Pour egg mixture into the greased 7-inch baking dish.

Cover dish with foil.

Select Bake mode.

Set time to 30 minutes and temperature 350 F then press START.

The air fryer display will prompt you to ADD FOOD once the temperature is reached then place the baking dish in the air fryer basket.

Serve and enjoy.

Almond Broccoli Muffins

Preparation Time: 10 minutes

Cooking Time: 30 minutes

Serve: 6

Ingredients

2 eggs

1 cup broccoli florets chopped

1 cup unsweetened almond milk

1 cup coconut flour

1 cup almond flour

1 tsp baking powder

2 tbsp nutritional yeast

1/2 tsp sea salt

Directions

Add all ingredients into the large bowl and mix until well combined.

Pour batter into the silicone muffin molds.

Select Bake mode.

Set time to 30 minutes and temperature 350 F then press START.

The air fryer display will prompt you to ADD FOOD once the temperature is reached then place muffin molds in the air fryer basket.

Serve and enjoy.

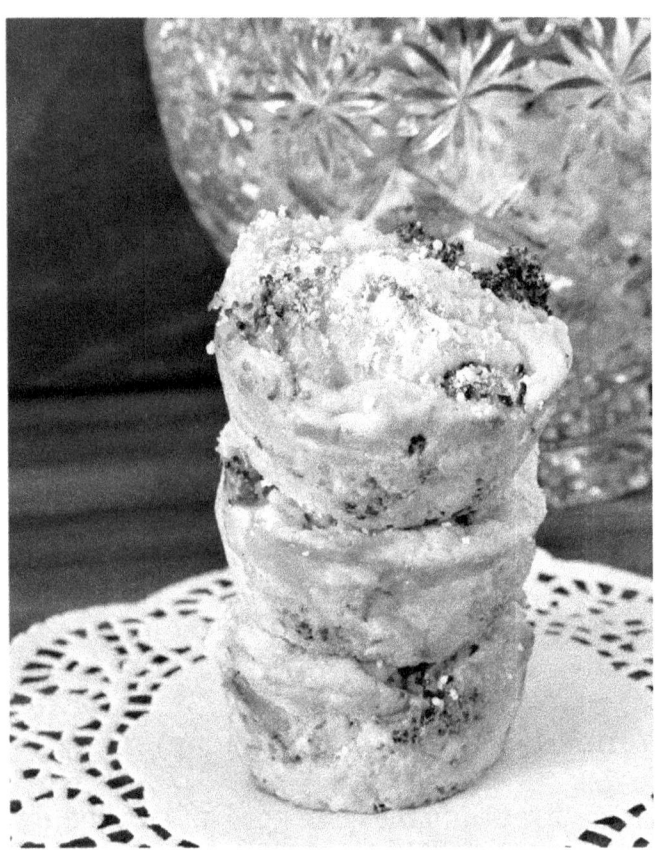

Italian Breakfast Frittata

Preparation Time: 10 minutes

Cooking Time: 30 minutes

Serve: 6

Ingredients

6 eggs

3/4 cup mozzarella cheese shredded

1/4 cup fresh basil chopped

1/2 cup tomatoes chopped

1 tsp Italian seasoning

2 tbsp water

Pepper

Salt

Directions

In a bowl, whisk eggs with water, 1/2 cheese, Italian seasoning, pepper, and salt.

Stir in remaining cheese, basil, and tomatoes.

Pour egg mixture into the greased 8-inch pie dish.

Cover dish with foil.

Select Bake mode.

Set time to 30 minutes and temperature 350 F then press START.

The air fryer display will prompt you to ADD FOOD once the temperature is reached then place the pie dish in the air fryer basket.

Serve and enjoy.

Fresh Herb Egg Cups

Preparation Time: 10 minutes

Cooking Time: 20 minutes

Serve: 6

Ingredients

6 eggs

1 tbsp fresh parsley chopped

1 tbsp chives chopped

1 tbsp fresh basil chopped

1 tbsp fresh cilantro chopped

1/4 cup mozzarella cheese grated

1 tbsp fresh dill chopped

Pepper

Salt

Directions

In a bowl, whisk eggs with pepper and salt.

Add remaining ingredients and stir well.

Pour egg mixture into the silicone muffin molds.

Select Bake mode.

Set time to 20 minutes and temperature 350 F then press START.

The air fryer display will prompt you to ADD FOOD once the temperature is reached then place muffin molds in the air fryer basket.

Serve and enjoy.

Feta Pepper Egg Muffins

Preparation Time: 10 minutes

Cooking Time: 20 minutes

Serve: 12

Ingredients

4 eggs

1/2 cup egg whites

1 tsp garlic powder

2 tbsp feta cheese crumbled

2 tbsp green onion chopped

4 fresh basil leaves chopped

1/4 cup unsweetened coconut milk

1 red bell pepper chopped

Pepper

Salt

Directions

In a bowl, whisk eggs, egg whites, milk, garlic powder, pepper, and salt.

Stir in cheese, bell pepper, green onion and basil.

Pour egg mixture into the silicone muffin molds.

Select Bake mode.

Set time to 20 minutes and temperature 350 F then press START.

The air fryer display will prompt you to ADD FOOD once the temperature is reached then place muffin molds in the air fryer basket.

Serve and enjoy.

Vanilla Raspberry Muffins

Preparation Time: 10 minutes

Cooking Time: 20 minutes

Serve: 12

Ingredients

3 eggs

1/2 cup raspberries

1/2 tsp vanilla

1/3 cup unsweetened almond milk

1/3 cup coconut oil melted

1 1/2 tsp baking powder

1/2 cup Swerve

2 1/2 cups almond flour

Directions

In a large bowl, mix almond flour, baking powder, and sweetener.

Stir in the coconut oil, vanilla, eggs, and almond milk.

Add raspberries and fold well.

Pour mixture into the silicone muffin molds.

Select Bake mode.

Set time to 20 minutes and temperature 350 F then press START.

The air fryer display will prompt you to ADD FOOD once the temperature is reached then place muffin molds in the air fryer basket.

Serve and enjoy.

Breakfast Bake Egg

Preparation Time: 10 minutes

Cooking Time: 15 minutes

Serve: 1

Ingredients

2 eggs

2 tbsp cheddar cheese shredded

2 tbsp half and half 1 tbsp parmesan cheese grated

1/2 tsp garlic powder

Pepper

Salt

Directions

In a small bowl, whisk eggs and a half and half.

Stir in cheddar cheese, parmesan cheese, pepper, and salt.

Pour egg mixture into the greased 8-ounce ramekin.

Select Bake mode.

Set time to 15 minutes and temperature 400 F then press START.

The air fryer display will prompt you to ADD FOOD once the temperature is reached then place the ramekin in the air fryer basket.

Serve and enjoy.

Easy Chicken Egg Cups

Preparation Time: 10 minutes

Cooking Time: 15 minutes

Serve: 12

Ingredients

10 eggs 1 cup chicken cooked and chopped

1/2 tsp garlic powder

1/4 tsp pepper

1 tsp sea salt

Directions

In a large bowl, whisk eggs with pepper and salt.

Add remaining ingredients and stir well.

Pour egg mixture into the silicone muffin molds.

Select Bake mode.

Set time to 15 minutes and temperature 400 F then press START.

The air fryer display will prompt you to ADD FOOD once the temperature is reached then place muffin molds in the air fryer basket.

Serve and enjoy.

Easy Breakfast Sausage

Preparation Time: 10 minutes

Cooking Time: 15 minutes

Serve: 6

Ingredients

2 lbs ground pork

1 tbsp dried parsley

1 tbsp Italian seasoning

2 tbsp olive oil

1 tsp paprika

1 tsp red pepper flakes

2 tsp salt

Directions

In a large bowl, combine together ground pork, paprika, red pepper flakes, parsley, Italian seasoning, olive oil, pepper, and salt.

Make small patties from the meat mixture.

Place the cooking tray in the air fryer basket.

Line air fryer basket with parchment paper.

Select Bake mode.

Set time to 15 minutes and temperature 375 F then press START.

The air fryer display will prompt you to ADD FOOD once the temperature is reached then place patties onto the parchment paper in the air fryer basket.

Serve and enjoy.

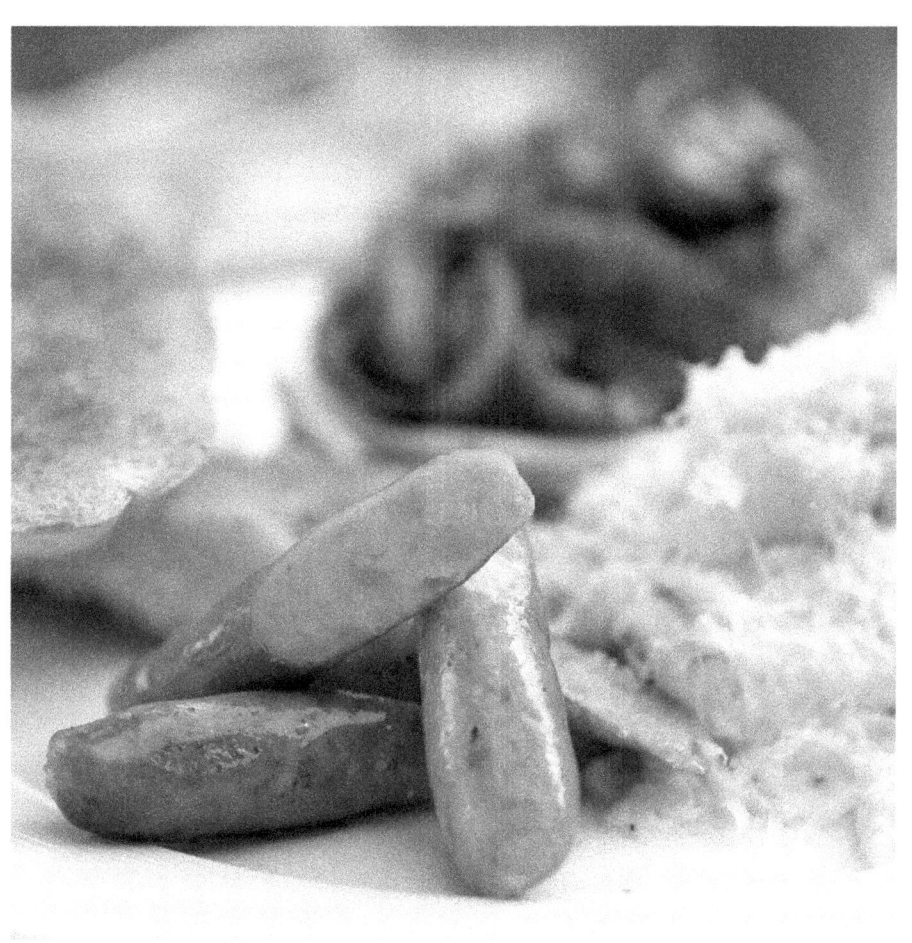

Zucchini Breakfast Casserole

Preparation Time: 10 minutes

Cooking Time: 50 minutes

Serve: 8

Ingredients

12 eggs

2 small zucchinis shredded

1 lb ground Italian sausage

3 tomatoes sliced

3 tbsp coconut flour

1/4 cup unsweetened almond milk

1/4 tsp pepper

1/2 tsp salt

Directions:

Cook sausage in a pan until lightly brown.

Transfer sausage to a large bowl.

Add coconut flour, milk, eggs, zucchini, pepper, and salt and mix well.

Add eggs and whisk until well combined.

Pour egg mixture into the greased casserole dish and top with tomato slices.

Cover dish with foil.

Select Bake mode.

Set time to 50 minutes and temperature 350 F then press START.

The air fryer display will prompt you to ADD FOOD once the temperature is reached then place a casserole dish in the air fryer basket.

Serve and enjoy.

Basil Cheese Zucchini Quiche

Preparation Time: 10 minutes

Cooking Time: 40 minutes

Serve: 6

Ingredients

3 eggs 1 cup mozzarella shredded

15 oz ricotta 1 onion chopped

2 medium zucchinis sliced

1/2 tsp dried oregano

1/2 tsp dried basil

1 tbsp olive oil

Black pepper

Salt

Directions

Heat oil in a pan over medium heat.

Add zucchini and sauté over low heat.

Add onion and cook for 10 minutes.

Add pepper and seasoning.

In a bowl, whisk eggs.

Stir in mozzarella, ricotta, onions, and zucchini.

Pour egg mixture into the greased pie dish.

Cover dish with foil.

Select Bake mode.

Set time to 30 minutes and temperature 350 F then press START.

The air fryer display will prompt you to ADD FOOD once the temperature is reached then place the pie dish in the air fryer basket.

Serve and enjoy.

Asparagus Quiche

Preparation Time: 10 minutes

Cooking Time: 30 minutes

Serve: 6

Ingredients

4 eggs

4 egg whites

1/4 cup water

8 oz asparagus cut into 1-inch pieces

2 tbsp feta cheese crumbled

1 cup cottage cheese

1/2 tsp dried thyme

1/4 tsp pepper

1/4 tsp salt

Directions

Add water into the large pot and bring to boil over high heat.

Add asparagus into the pot and cook for 2 minutes.

Drain well.

In a large bowl, whisk egg whites, eggs, cottage cheese, thyme, water, pepper, and salt.

Pour egg mixture into the greased baking dish.

Add asparagus pieces into the egg mixture and top with feta cheese.

Cover dish with foil.

Select Bake mode.

Set time to 30 minutes and temperature 375 F then press START.

The air fryer display will prompt you to ADD FOOD once the temperature is reached then place the baking dish in the air fryer basket.

Slice and serve.

Moist Pumpkin Muffins

Preparation Time: 10 minutes

Cooking Time: 15 minutes

Serve: 20

Ingredients

2 scoops vanilla protein powder

1/2 cup almond flour

1/2 cup coconut oil

1/2 cup pumpkin puree

1/2 cup almond butter

1 tbsp cinnamon

1 tsp baking powder

Directions

In a large bowl, mix together all dry ingredients.

Add wet ingredients into the dry ingredients and mix until well combined.

Pour batter into the silicone muffin molds.

Select Bake mode.

Set time to 15 minutes and temperature 350 F then press START.

The air fryer display will prompt you to ADD FOOD once the temperature is reached then place muffin molds in the air fryer basket.

Serve and enjoy.

Healthy Zucchini Gratin

Preparation Time: 10 minutes

Cooking Time: 30 minutes

Serve: 4

Ingredients

1 egg lightly beaten

3 medium zucchinis sliced

1/2 cup nutritional yeast

1/4 cup unsweetened almond milk

1 tbsp Dijon mustard

1 tsp sea salt

Directions

Arrange zucchini slices in the oven-safe casserole dish.

In a saucepan, heat almond milk over low heat and stir in Dijon mustard, nutritional yeast, and sea salt.

Add egg and whisk well.

Pour sauce over zucchini slices.

Cover dish with foil.

Select Bake mode.

Set time to 30 minutes and temperature 400 F then press START.

The air fryer display will prompt you to ADD FOOD once the temperature is reached then place a casserole dish in the air fryer basket.

Serve and enjoy.

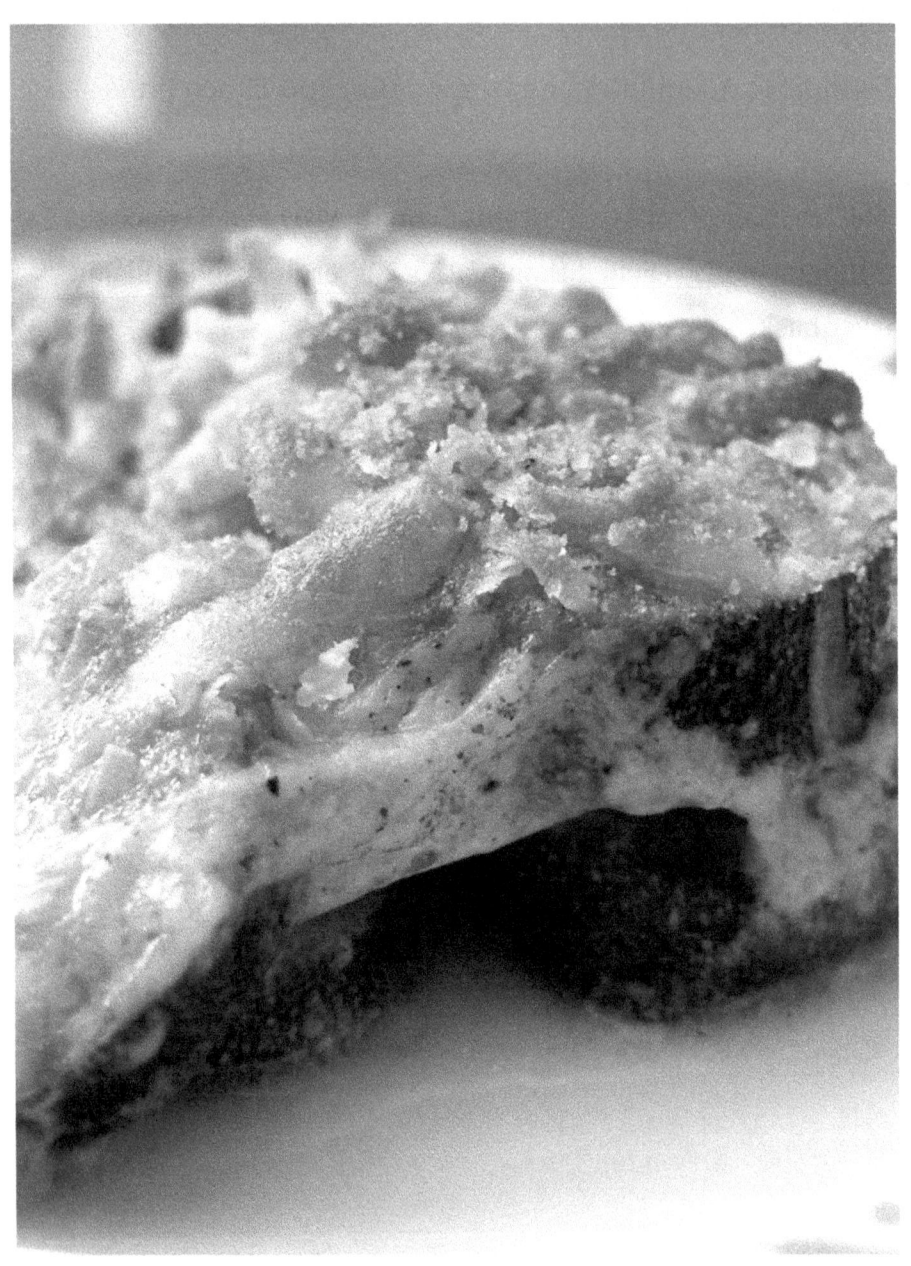

Artichoke Quiche

Preparation Time: 10 minutes

Cooking Time: 40 minutes

Serve: 4

Ingredients

3 eggs

1 cup artichoke hearts chopped

1 cup mushrooms sliced

1 small onion chopped

3 garlic cloves minced

1/2 cup cottage cheese fat-free

10 oz spinach frozen

1/2 tsp olive oil

Pepper

Salt

Directions

Heat oil in a pan over medium heat.

Add onion, mushrooms, garlic, and spinach and sauté for a minute.

In a bowl add cheese, artichoke hearts, eggs, pepper, and salt mix well.

Add sautéed vegetable mixture to the bowl and mix well.

Pour egg mixture into the greased baking dish.

Cover dish with foil.

Select Bake mode.

Set time to 40 minutes and temperature 350 F then press START.

The air fryer display will prompt you to ADD FOOD once the temperature is reached then place the baking dish in the air fryer basket.

Serve and enjoy.

Tomato Feta Frittata

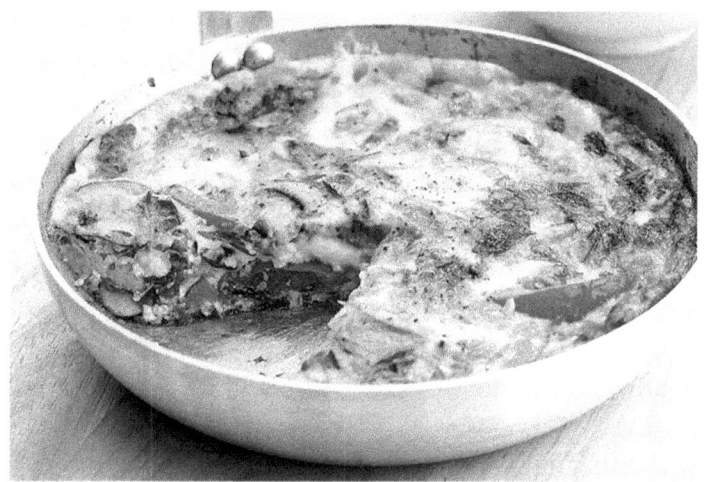

Preparation Time: 10 minutes

Cooking Time: 7 minutes

Serve: 2

Ingredients

6 eggs

2/3 cup feta cheese crumbled

1 small onion chopped

1 tbsp fresh chives chopped

1 tbsp olive oil 1 tbsp fresh basil chopped

3 oz cherry tomatoes halved

Pepper

Salt

Directions

Heat oil in a pan over medium-high heat.

Add onion and sauté until lightly browned.

Remove from heat.

In a bowl, whisk eggs, basil, chives, pepper, and salt.

Stir in sauteed onion, cherry tomatoes, and crumbled cheese.

Pour egg mixture into the greased baking dish.

Select Broil mode.

Set time to 7 minutes and temperature 400 F then press START.

The air fryer display will prompt you to ADD FOOD once the temperature is reached then place the baking dish in the air fryer basket.

Serve and enjoy.

Blueberry Cream Cheese Toasts

Prep + Cook Time: 15 minutes

Servings: 2

INGREDIENTS

2 eggs beaten

4 bread slices

1 tbsp sugar

1 ½ cups corn flakes

⅓ cup milk

¼ tsp ground nutmeg

4 tbsp whipped cream cheese

1 tbsp blueberry preserves

DIRECTIONS

Preheat air fryer to 390 F.

In a bowl, mix sugar, eggs, nutmeg, and milk.

In a separate bowl, whisk the cream cheese and blueberry preserves.

Spread the blueberry mixture on 2 bread slices.

Cover with the remaining 2 slices to make sandwiches.

Dip in the egg mixture, then thoroughly coat in cornflakes.

Lay the sandwiches in the air fryer's basket and cook for 8 minutes, flipping once.

Serve immediately.

Onion & Cheddar Omelet

Prep + Cook Time: 20 minutes

2 Servings

INGREDIENTS

4 eggs

3 tbsp cheddar cheese grated

1 tsp soy sauce

½ onion sliced

DIRECTIONS

Preheat air fryer to 350 F.

Whisk the eggs with soy sauce and mix in onion.

Pour the egg mixture into a greased baking pan and place it in the fryer's basket.

Bake for 12-14 minutes.

Top with the grated cheddar cheese and serve right away.

Best served with a tomato salad or freshly chopped scallions.

Spicy Egg & Bacon Tortilla Wraps

Prep + Cook Time: 15 minutes

3 Servings

INGREDIENTS

3 flour tortillas 2 eggs scrambled

3 slices bacon cut into strips

3 tbsp salsa

3 tbsp cream cheese

1 cup Pepper Jack cheese grated

DIRECTIONS

Preheat air fryer to 390 F.

Spread the cream cheese on the tortillas.

Add the eggs and bacon and top with salsa.

Scatter over the grated cheese and roll up tightly.

Place in the fryer's basket and AirFry for 10 minutes or until golden.

Cut in half and serve warm.

Turkey & Mushroom Sandwich

Prep + Cook Time: 10 minutes

1 Serving

INGREDIENTS

⅓ cup leftover turkey shredded

⅓ cup sliced mushrooms sauteed

½ tbsp butter softened

2 tomato slices

½ tsp red pepper flakes

Salt and black pepper to taste

1 hamburger bun halved

DIRECTIONS

Preheat air fryer to 350 F.

Brush the bottom half with butter and top with shredded turkey.

Arrange mushroom slices on top of the turkey.

Cover with tomato slices and sprinkle with salt, black pepper, and red flakes.

Top with the other bun half and AirFry in the fryer for 5-8 minutes until crispy.

Grilled Tofu Sandwich with Cabbage

Prep + Cook Time: 20 minutes

1 Serving

INGREDIENTS

2 slices of bread

1 slice tofu

1-inch thick

¼ cup red cabbage shredded

2 tsp olive oil

¼ tsp vinegar

Salt and black pepper to taste

DIRECTIONS

Preheat air fryer to 350 F.

Add the bread slices to the air fryer basket and toast for 3 minutes; set aside.

Brush the tofu with some olive oil and place in the air fryer to Bake for 5 minutes on each side.

Mix the cabbage, remaining olive oil, and vinegar.

Season with salt.

Place the tofu on top of one bread slice, place the cabbage over, and top with the other bread slice.

Serve with cream cheese-mustard dip.

Omelet Bread Cups

Prep + Cook Time: 25 minutes

4 Servings

INGREDIENTS

4 crusty rolls

5 eggs beaten

½ tsp thyme dried

3 strips cooked bacon chopped

2 tbsp heavy cream

4 Gouda cheese thin slices

DIRECTIONS

Preheat air fryer to 330 F.

Cut the tops off the rolls and remove the inside with your fingers.

Line the rolls with a slice of cheese and press down, so the cheese conforms to the inside of the roll.

In a bowl, mix the eggs, heavy cream, bacon, and thyme.

Stuff the rolls with the egg mixture.

Lay them in the greased air fryer's basket and bake for 8-10 minutes or until the eggs become puffy, and the roll shows a golden-brown texture.

Remove and serve immediately.

Prosciutto, Mozzarella & Eggs in a Cup

Prep + Cook Time: 20 minutes

2 Servings

INGREDIENTS

2 bread slices

2 prosciutto slices chopped

2 eggs

4 tomato slices

¼ tsp balsamic vinegar

2 tbsp mozzarella cheese grated

¼ tsp maple syrup

2 tbsp mayonnaise

Salt and black pepper to taste

Cooking spray

DIRECTIONS

Preheat air fryer to 350 F.

Grease 2 ramekins with cooking spray.

Place one bread slice on the bottom of each ramekin.

Place 2 tomato slices on top and divide mozzarella cheese between the ramekins.

Crack the eggs over the mozzarella cheese.

Drizzle with maple syrup and balsamic vinegar.

Season with salt and pepper and Bake for 10 minutes in the fryer.

Top with mayonnaise and serve.

Crustless Mediterranean Quiche

Prep + Cook Time: 40 minutes

2 Servings

INGREDIENTS

4 eggs ½ cup tomatoes chopped

1 cup feta cheese crumbled

½ tbsp fresh basil chopped

½ tbsp fresh oregano chopped

¼ cup Kalamata olives sliced

¼ cup onions chopped

½ cup milk

Salt and black pepper to taste

DIRECTIONS

Preheat air fryer to 340 F.

Beat the eggs along with the milk, salt, and pepper.

Stir in all the remaining ingredients.

Pour the egg mixture into a greased baking pan that fits in your air fryer and place in the fryer.

Bake for 30 minutes or until lightly golden.

Serve warm with a green salad.

Air Fried Italian Calzone

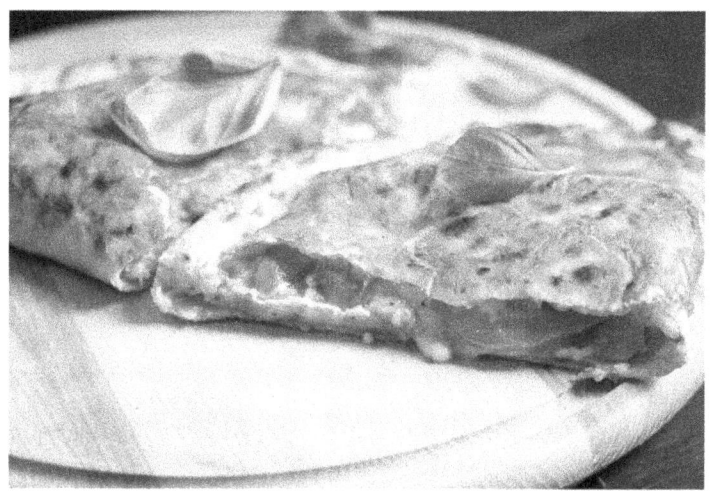

Prep + Cook Time: 20 minutes

4 Servings

INGREDIENTS

1 pizza dough

4 oz cheddar cheese grated

1 oz mozzarella cheese grated

1 oz bacon diced

2 cups cooked turkey shredded

1 egg beaten

4 tbsp tomato paste

½ tsp dried basil

½ tsp dried oregano

Salt and black pepper to taste

DIRECTIONS

Preheat air fryer to 350 F.

Divide the pizza dough into 4 equal pieces, so you have the dough for 4 pizza crusts.

Combine the tomato paste, basil, and oregano in a small bowl.

Brush the mixture onto the crusts; make sure not to go all the way and avoid brushing near the edges of each crust.

Scatter half of the turkey on top and season with salt and pepper.

Top with bacon, mozzarella and cheddar cheeses.

Brush the edges with the beaten egg.

Fold the crusts and seal with a fork.

Bake for 10-12 minutes until puffed and golden, turning over halfway through the cooking time.

Serve.

Italian Sausage Patties

Prep + Cook Time: 20 minutes

4 Servings

INGREDIENTS

1 lb ground Italian sausage

¼ cup breadcrumbs

1 tsp red pepper flakes

Salt and black pepper to taste

¼ tsp garlic powder

1 egg beaten

DIRECTIONS

Preheat air fryer to 350 F.

Combine all the ingredients in a large bowl.

Make patties out of the mixture and arrange them on a greased baking sheet.

Add to the fryer and AirFry for 15 minutes, flipping once.

Brioche Toast with Chocolate

Prep + Cook Time: 15 minutes

2 Servings

INGREDIENTS

4 slices of brioche

3 eggs

4 tbsp butter

6 oz milk chocolate broken into chunks

½ cup heavy cream

1 tsp vanilla extract

½ cup maple syrup

½ tsp salt

DIRECTIONS

Preheat air fryer to 350 F.

Beat the eggs with heavy cream, salt, and vanilla in a small bowl.

Dip the brioche slices in the egg mixture and AirFry in the greased fryer for 7-8 minutes in total, shaking once or twice.

Melt the chocolate and butter in the microwave for 60-90 seconds, remove, and whisk with a fork until well combined.

Let cool slightly.

When the brioches are ready, remove, and dip in the chocolate-butter mixture.

Serve with a cup of tea and enjoy!

Breakfast Egg Muffins with Shrimp

Prep + Cook Time: 35 minutes

4 Servings

INGREDIENTS

4 eggs beaten

2 tbsp olive oil

½ small red bell pepper finely diced

1 garlic clove minced

4 oz shrimp cooked chopped

4 tsp ricotta cheese crumbled

1 tsp dry dill

Salt and black pepper to taste

DIRECTIONS

Preheat air fryer to 360 F.

Warm the olive oil in a skillet over medium heat.

Sauté the bell pepper and garlic until the pepper is soft, then add the shrimp.

Season with dill, salt, and pepper and cook for about 5 minutes.

Remove from the heat and mix in the eggs.

Grease 4 ramekins with cooking spray.

Divide the mixture between the ramekins.

Place them in the fryer and cook for 6 minutes.

Remove and stir the mixture.

Sprinkle with ricotta and return to the fryer.

Cook for 5 minutes until the eggs are set, and the top is lightly browned.

Let sit for 2 minutes, invert on a plate, while warm and serve.

Kiwi Muffins with Pecans

Prep + Cook Time: 25 minutes

4 Servings

INGREDIENTS

1 cup flour 1 kiwi mashed

¼ cup powdered sugar

1 tsp milk 1 tbsp pecans chopped

½ tsp baking powder

¼ cup oats

¼ cup butter room temperature

DIRECTIONS

Preheat air fryer to 350 F.

Place the sugar, pecans, kiwi, and butter in a bowl and mix well.

In another bowl, mix the flour, baking powder, and oats and stir well.

Combine the two mixtures and stir in the milk.

Pour the batter into a greased muffin tin that fits in the fryer and Bake for 15 minutes.

Remove to a wire rack and leave to cool for a few minutes before removing from the muffin tin.

Enjoy!

Hearty Banana Pastry

Prep + Cook Time: 20 minutes

2 Servings

INGREDIENTS

3 bananas sliced

3 tbsp honey

2 puff pastry sheets cut into thin strips

1 cup fresh berries to serve

DIRECTIONS

Preheat air fryer to 340 F.

Place the banana slices into a greased baking dish.

Cover with pastry strips and drizzle with honey.

Bake in the air fryer for 12 minutes until golden.

Serve with berries.

Mango Bread

Prep + Cook Time: 30 minutes

6 Servings

INGREDIENTS

½ cup butter melted

1 egg lightly beaten

½ cup brown sugar

1 tsp vanilla extract

3 ripe mangoes mashed

1 ½ cups flour

1 tsp baking powder

½ tsp grated nutmeg

½ tsp ground cinnamon

DIRECTIONS

Line a loaf tin with baking paper.

In a bowl, whisk melted butter, egg, sugar, vanilla, and mangoes.

Sift in flour, baking powder, nutmeg, and ground cinnamon and stir without overmixing.

Pour the batter into the tin and place it in the air fryer.

Bake for 18-20 minutes at 330 F.

Let cool before slicing and serve.

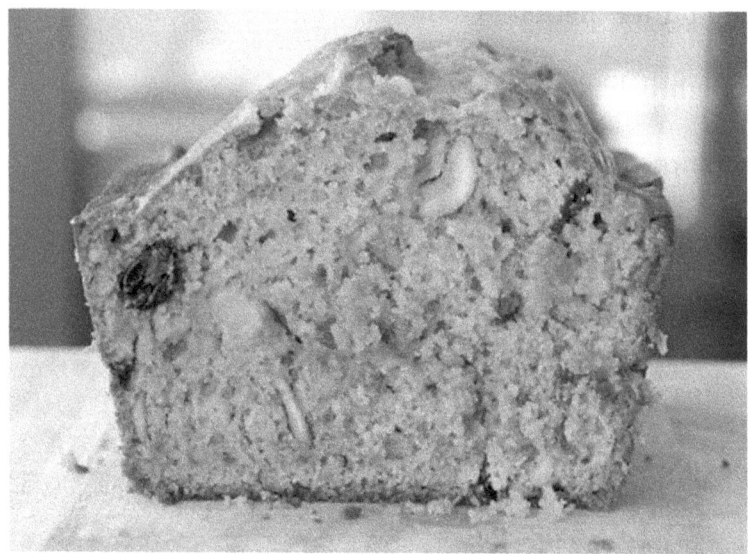

Pumpkin & Sultanas' Bread

Prep + Cook Time: 30 minutes + cooling time

6 Servings

INGREDIENTS

1 cup pumpkin peeled and shredded

1 cup flour

1 tsp ground nutmeg

½ tsp salt

¼ tsp baking powder

2 eggs

½ cup sugar

¼ cup milk

2 tbsp butter melted

½ tsp vanilla extract

2 tbsp sultanas soaked

1 tbsp honey

1 tbsp canola oil

DIRECTIONS

Preheat air fryer to 350 F.

In a bowl, beat the eggs and add in pumpkin, sugar, milk, canola oil, sultanas, and vanilla.

In a separate bowl, sift the flour and mix in nutmeg, salt, butter, and baking powder.

Combine the 2 mixtures and stir until a thick cake mixture forms.

Spoon the batter into a greased baking dish and place it in the air fryer.

Bake for 25 minutes until a toothpick inserted in the center comes out clean and dry.

Remove to a wire rack to cool completely.

Drizzle with honey and serve.

French Toast with Vanilla Filling

Prep + Cook Time: 15 minutes

3 Servings

INGREDIENTS

6 slices white bread

2 eggs

¼ cup heavy cream

⅓ cup sugar mixed with 1 tsp ground cinnamon

6 tbsp caramel

1 tsp vanilla extract

Cooking spray

DIRECTIONS

In a bowl, whisk eggs, and heavy cream.

Dip each piece of bread into the egg mixture.

Coat the bread with sugar and cinnamon mixture.

On a clean board, lay the coated slices and spread three of the slices with about 2 tbsp of caramel each around the center.

Place the remaining three slices on top to form three sandwiches.

Spray the air fryer basket with some cooking spray.

Arrange the sandwiches into the fryer and cook for 10 minutes at 340 F, turning once.

Greek-Style Frittata

Prep + Cook Time: 30 minutes

4 Servings

INGREDIENTS

5 eggs

1 cup baby spinach

½ cup grape tomatoes halved

½ cup feta cheese crumbled

10 Kalamata olives sliced

Salt and black pepper to taste

2 tbsp fresh parsley chopped

DIRECTIONS

Preheat air fryer to 360 F.

Beat the eggs, salt, and pepper in a bowl, combining well before adding the spinach and stirring until all is mixed.

Pour half the mixture into a greased baking pan.

On top of the mixture, add half of the tomatoes, olives, and feta.

Cover the pan with foil, making sure to close it tightly around the edges, then place the pan in the air fryer and cook for 12 minutes.

Remove the foil and cook for an additional 5-7 minutes, until the eggs are fully cooked.

Place the finished frittata on a serving plate and repeat the above instructions for the remainder of the ingredients.

Decorate with parsley and cut into wedges. Serve hot or at room temperature.

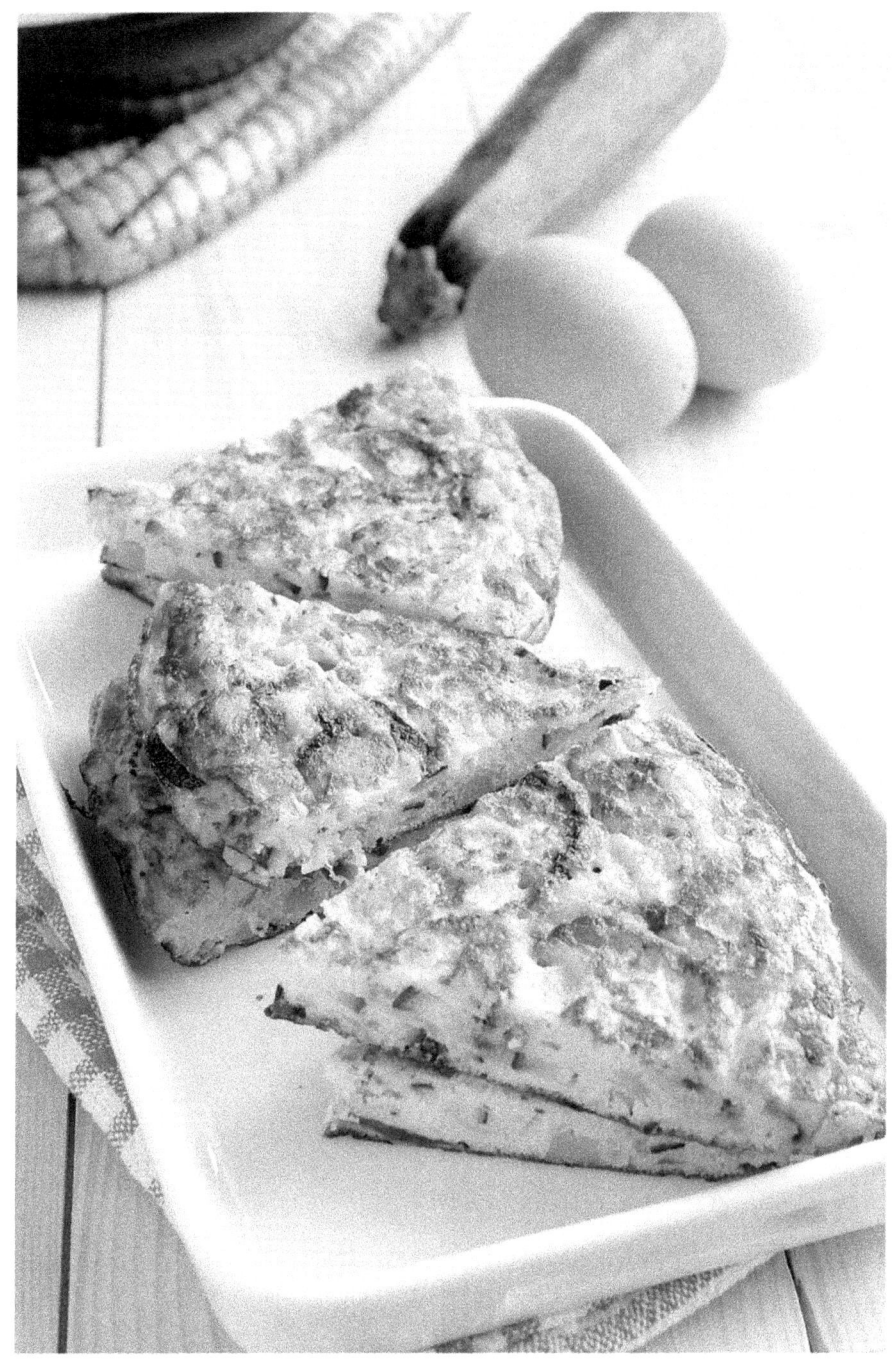

Morning Potato Skins

Prep + Cook Time: 35 minutes

4 Servings

INGREDIENTS

4 eggs 2 large russet potatoes scrubbed

1 tbsp olive oil

2 tbsp cooked bacon chopped

1 cup cheddar cheese shredded

1 tbsp chopped chives

¼ tsp red pepper flakes

Salt and black pepper to taste

DIRECTIONS

Preheat air fryer to 360 F.

Using a fork, poke holes in all sides of the potatoes, then cook them in the microwave on high for 5 minutes.

Flip the potatoes and cook in the microwave for another 3-5 minutes.

Test with a fork to make sure they are tender.

Halve the potatoes lengthwise and scoop out most of the 'meat,' leaving enough potato, so the sides of the 'boat' don't collapse.

Coat the skin side of the potatoes with olive oil, salt, and pepper for taste.

Arrange the potatoes, skin down, in the lightly greased air fryer basket.

Crack an egg and put it in the scooped potato, one egg for each half.

Divide the bacon and cheddar cheese between the potatoes and sprinkle with salt and pepper.

For a runny yolk, air fry for 5-6 minutes, and for a solid yolk, air fry for 7-10 minutes.

Sprinkle with red pepper flakes and chives.

Serve immediately.

Buttered Eggs in Hole

Prep + Cook Time: 15 minutes

2 Servings

INGREDIENTS

2 bread slices

2 eggs

Salt and black pepper to taste

2 tbsp butter

DIRECTIONS

Preheat air fryer to 360 F.

Place a heatproof bowl in the fryer's basket and brush with butter.

Make a hole in the middle of the bread slices with a bread knife and place on the heatproof bowl in 2 batches.

Crack an egg into the center of each hole; season.

Bake in the air fryer for 4 minutes.

Turn the bread with a spatula and cook for another 4 minutes. Serve warm.

Loaded Egg Pepper Rings

Prep + Cook Time: 15 minutes

4 Servings

INGREDIENTS

4 eggs

1 bell pepper cut into four

¾-inch rings 5 cherry tomatoes halved

Salt and black pepper to taste

DIRECTIONS

Preheat air fryer to 360 F.

Put the bell pepper rings in a greased baking pan and crack an egg into each one.

Season with salt and pepper.

Top with the halved cherry tomatoes.

Put the pan into the air fryer and air fry for 6-9 minutes, or until the eggs are have set.

Serve and enjoy!

Chili Hash Browns

Prep + Cook Time: 25 minutes + cooling time

4 Servings

INGREDIENTS

1 lb potatoes, peeled and shredded

Salt and black pepper to taste

1 tsp garlic powder

1 tsp chili flakes 1 tsp onion powder

1 egg beaten

1 tbsp olive oil

Cooking spray

DIRECTIONS

Heat olive oil in a skillet over medium heat and sauté potatoes for 10 minutes.

Transfer to a bowl.

After they have cooled, add in the egg, pepper, salt, chili flakes, onion powder, and garlic powder and mix well.

On a flat plate, spread the mixture and pat it firmly with your fingers.

Refrigerate for 20 minutes.

Preheat air fryer to 350 F.

Shape the cooled into patties.

Grease the air fryer basket with cooking spray and arrange the patties in.

Cook for 12 minutes on AirFry mode, flipping once.

Serve warm.

Japanese-Style Omelet

Prep + Cook Time: 20 minutes

1 Serving

INGREDIENTS

1 cup cubed tofu

3 whole eggs

Salt and black pepper to taste

¼ tsp ground coriander

¼ tsp cumin

1 tsp soy sauce

1 tbsp green onions chopped

¼ onion chopped

DIRECTIONS

In a bowl, mix eggs, onion, soy sauce, coriander, cumin, black pepper, and salt.

 Add in cubed tofu and pour the mixture into a greased baking tray.

Place in the air fryer and Bake for 8 minutes at 400 F.

When ready, remove, and sprinkle with green onions to serve.

Baked Kale Omelet

Prep + Cook Time: 15 minutes

2 Servings

INGREDIENTS

5 eggs

3 tbsp cottage cheese crumbled

1 cup kale chopped

½ tbsp fresh basil chopped

½ tbsp fresh parsley chopped

Salt and black pepper to taste

DIRECTIONS

Beat the eggs, salt, and pepper in a bowl.

Stir in the rest of the ingredients.

Pour the mixture into a greased baking pan and fit in the air fryer.

Bake for 10 minutes at 330 F until slightly golden and set.

Baked Avocado with Eggs & Cilantro

Prep + Cook Time: 10 minutes

1 Serving

INGREDIENTS

1 ripe avocado pitted and halved

2 eggs

Salt and black pepper to taste

1 tsp fresh cilantro chopped

DIRECTIONS

Preheat air fryer to 400 F.

Crack one egg into each avocado half and place in the air fryer.

Bake for 8-12 minutes until the eggs are cooked through.

Sprinkle with salt and black pepper and let cool slightly.

Top with freshly chopped cilantro and serve warm.

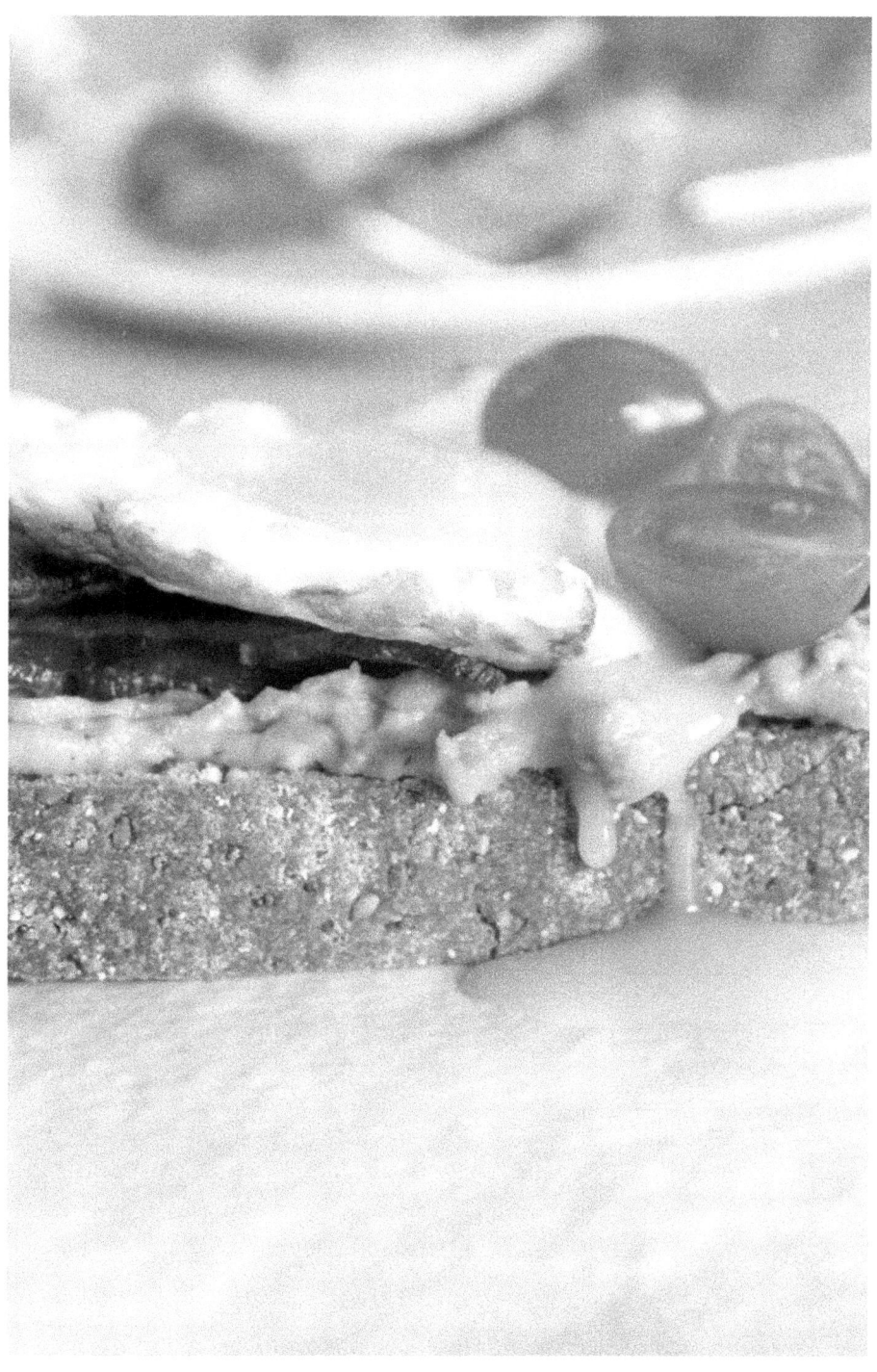

www.ingramcontent.com/pod-product-compliance
Lightning Source LLC
Chambersburg PA
CBHW071109030426
42336CB00013BA/2007